Leukemia in Our School

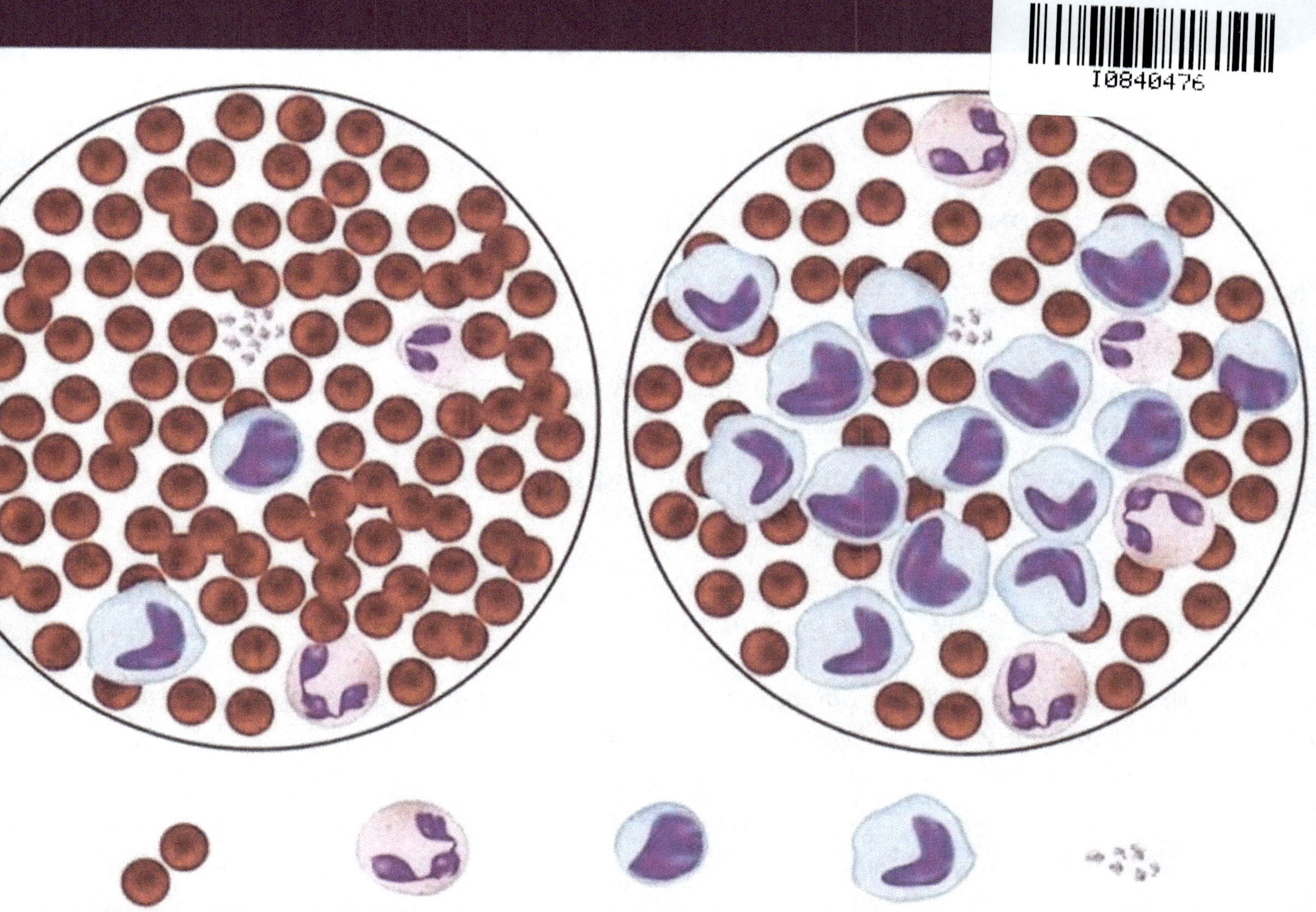

By Jonathan Ritchie

Text by Jonathan Ritchie with contributions from Abigail Mapel.

Additional support and mentorship from Jacob Gorczyca.

Special thanks to Officer Mark Smilek.

Cover image from Creative Biolabs In Vitro Diagnostics.
Image of cancer statistics from *CA: A Cancer Journal for Clinicians* published by Wiley Periodicals LLC on behalf of American Cancer Society
Some images may be subject to copyright

ISBN 978-1-716-40159-6

Grow a Generation
Sewickley, PA 15143
www.growageneration.com

Any and all profits from the sale of this book benefit The Hillman Cancer Center

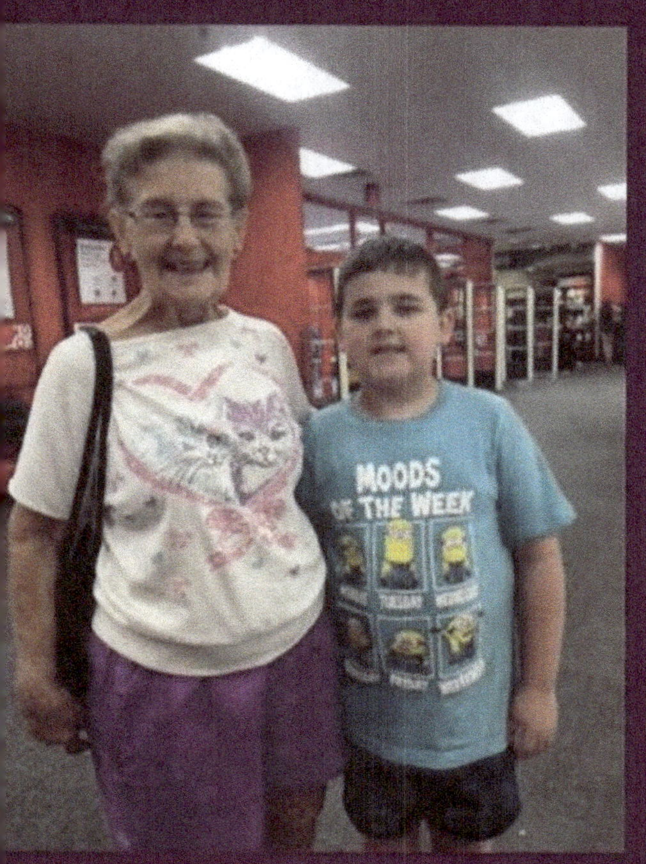

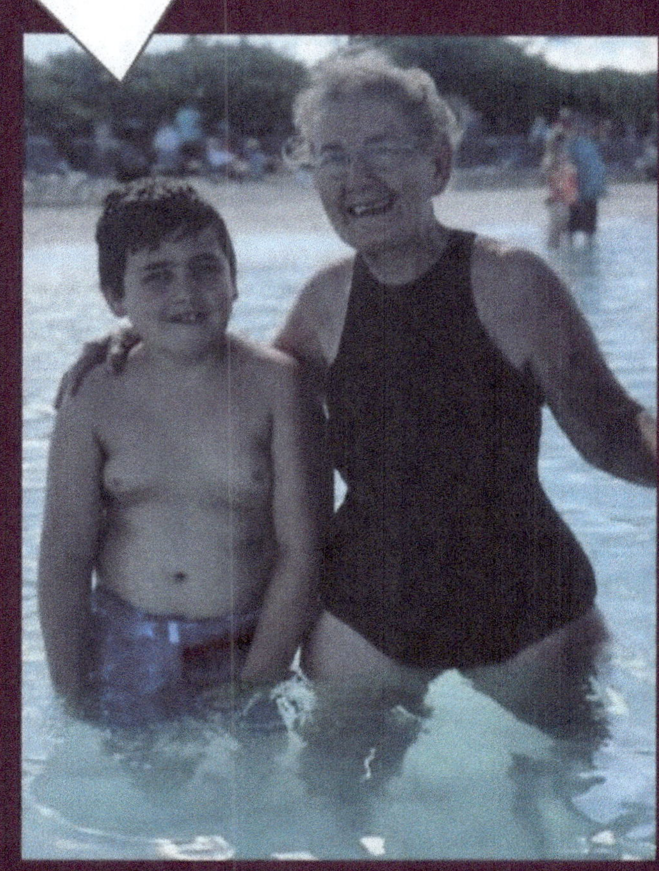

She liked to have fun, travel, and come to my soccer games. She also loved cooking good food for her family and helping me get on and off the bus!

I go to a school called Baden Academy. We have a
school resource officer there named Officer Mark!
He is always friendly and helpful, just like my
Great Gram. He does an excellent job keeping
everyone safe.

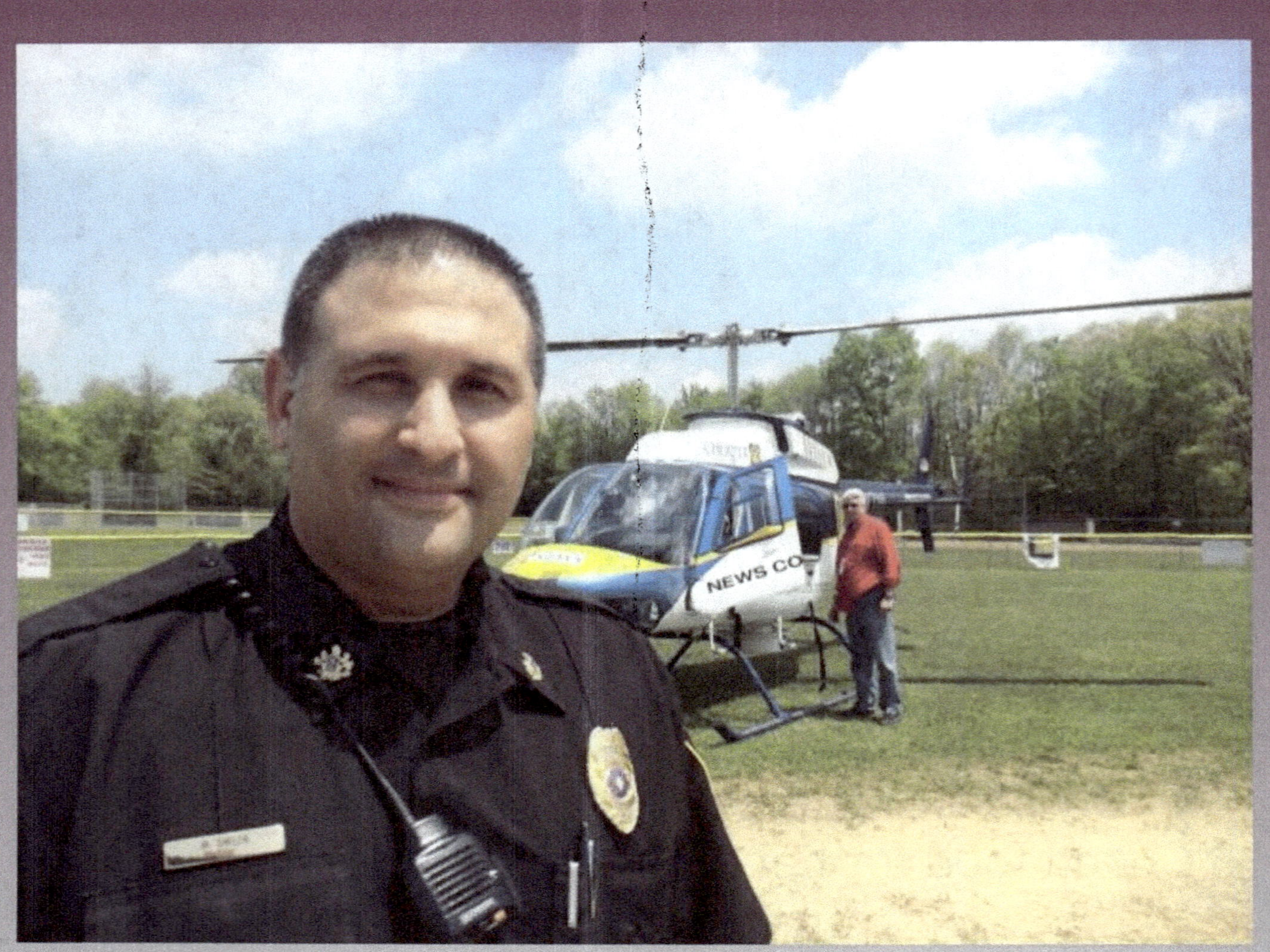

Great Gram continued helping until she felt really tired and started losing a lot of weight. She still did as much as she could to spend time with our family. In 2020 we celebrated her birthday and took a trip to Kinzua. Shortly after, she was admitted to the hospital.

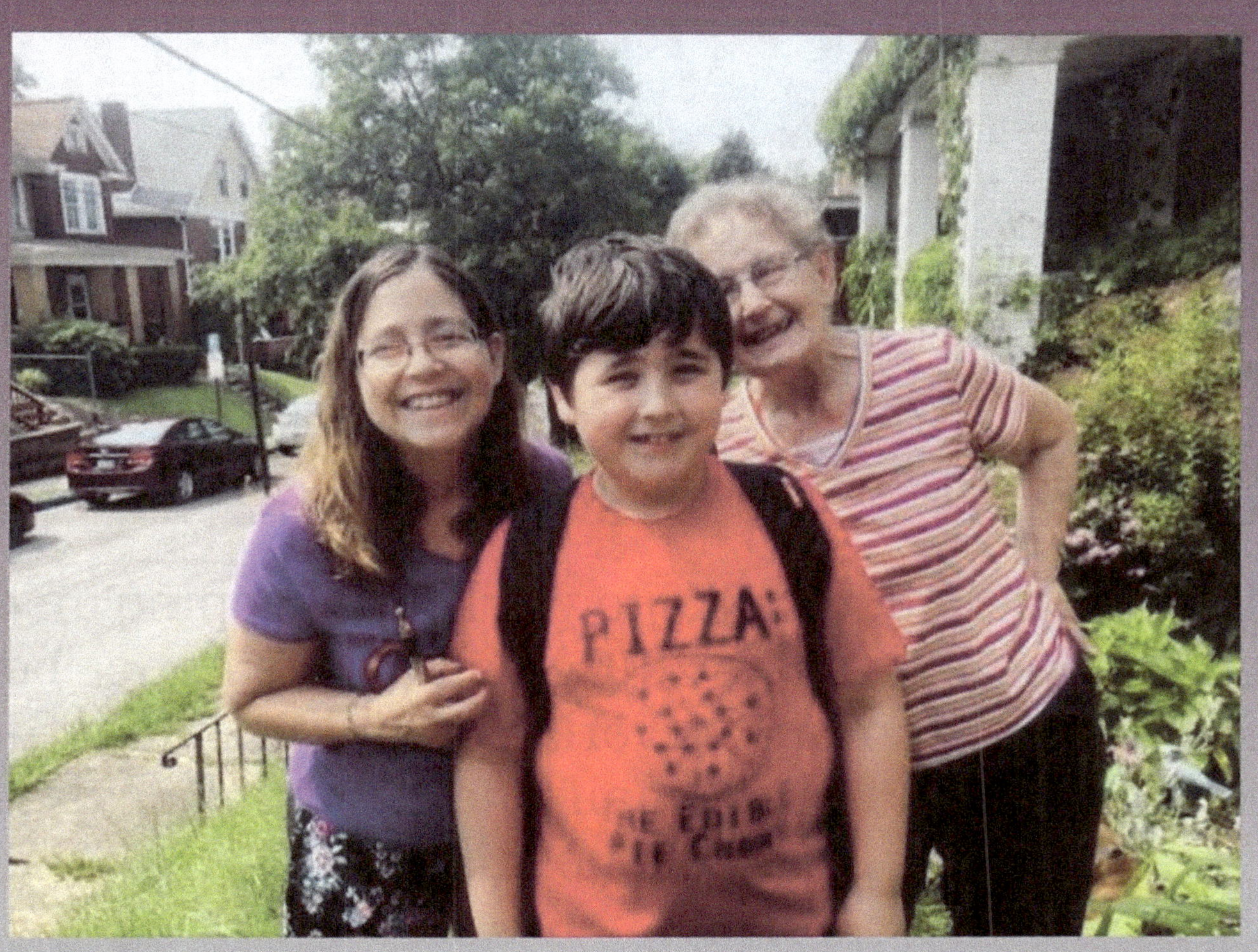

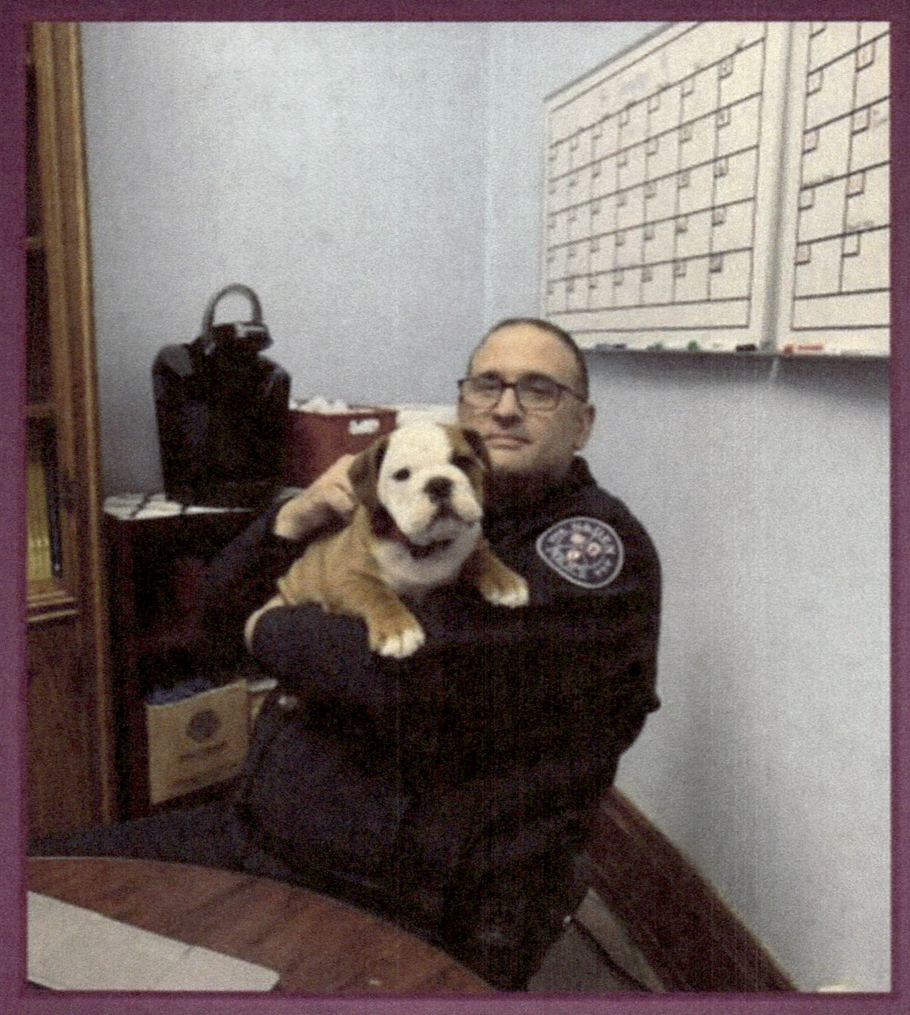

Officer Mark kept coming to work and keeping an eye on everyone, but in late 2016 he started to notice bone pain. He had to continue working, but knew that there was something wrong. Finally, he knew it was time to go to the hospital.

They were both diagnosed with leukemia. Officer Mark was diagnosed with ALL in May of 2017. It is a pediatric leukemia that rarely happens in adults (only about 7,000 cases per year). Great Gram was diagnosed at the end June, 2020 with AML. It is an aggressive type of cancer with only a 20% survival rate in people over 20 years old.

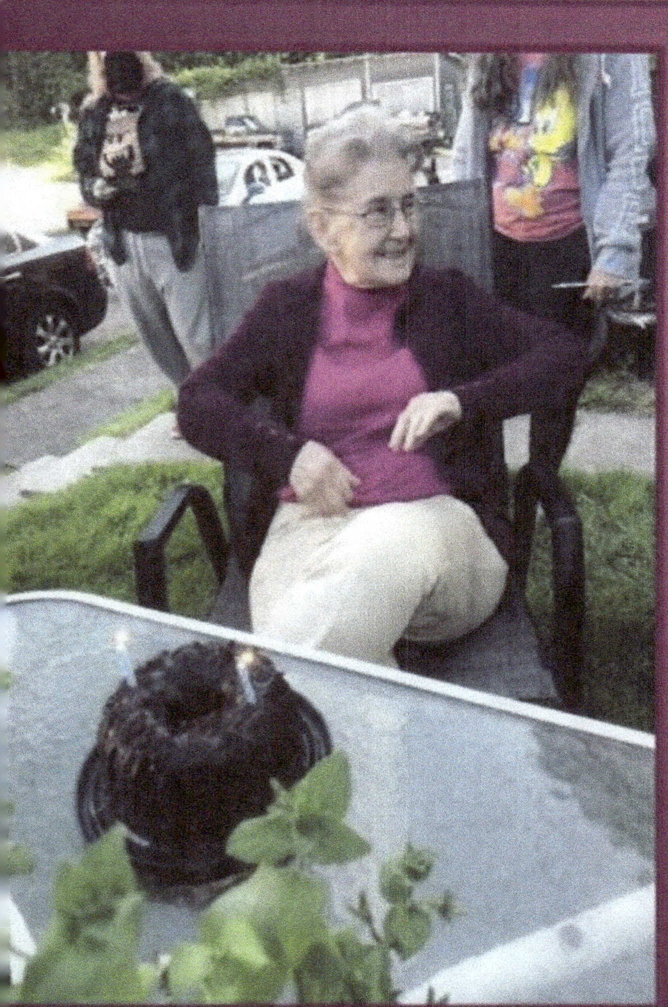

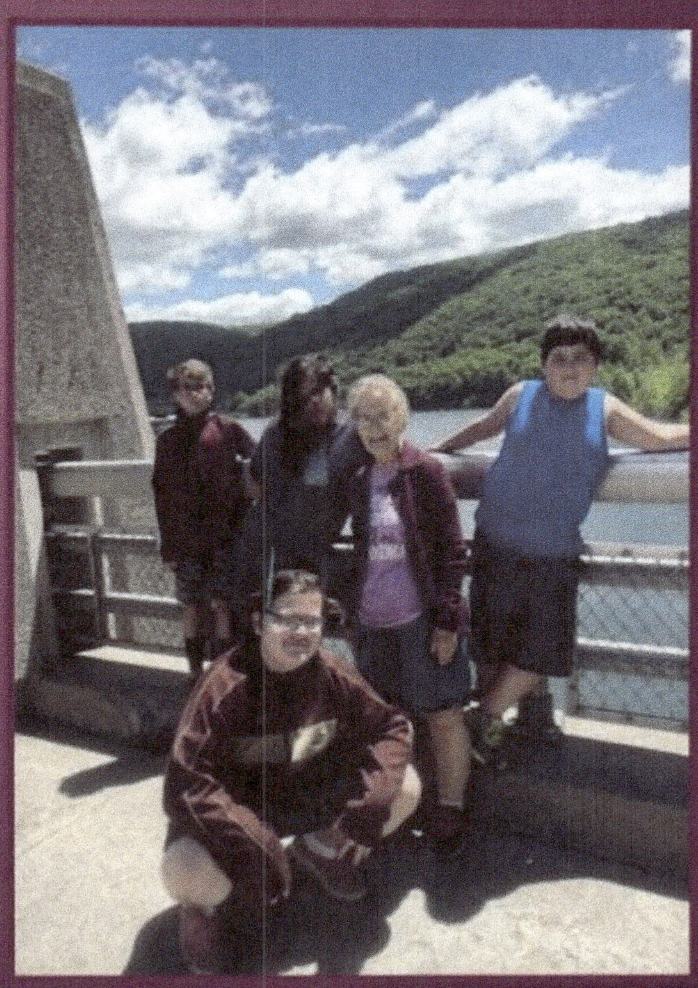

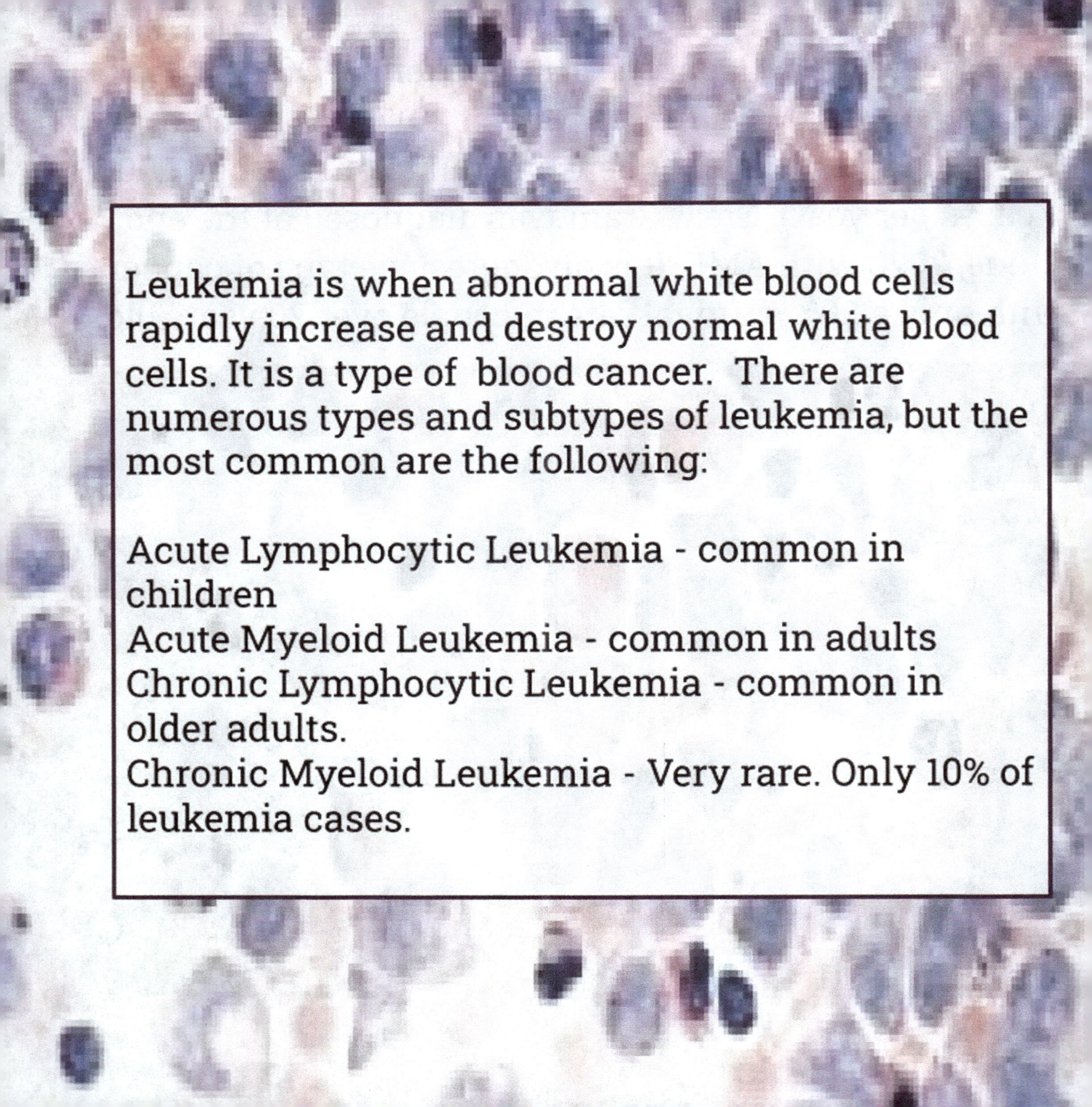

Leukemia is when abnormal white blood cells rapidly increase and destroy normal white blood cells. It is a type of blood cancer. There are numerous types and subtypes of leukemia, but the most common are the following:

Acute Lymphocytic Leukemia - common in children
Acute Myeloid Leukemia - common in adults
Chronic Lymphocytic Leukemia - common in older adults.
Chronic Myeloid Leukemia - Very rare. Only 10% of leukemia cases.

Leukemia Symptoms differ depending on the patient and the type but can include:

Coughing or chest pain
Fever or chills
Frequent infections
Bleeding
Rash
Loss of appetite or nausea
Night sweats
Persistent weakness and fatigue
Shortness of breath
Swollen, painless lymph nodes in the neck, armpits, or groin

Estimated New Cases, 2022

Males			Females	
Prostate	268,490	27%	Breast	287,850
Lung & bronchus	117,910	12%	Lung & bronchus	118,830
Colon & rectum	80,690	8%	Colon & rectum	70,340
Urinary bladder	61,700	6%	Uterine corpus	65,950
Melanoma of the skin	57,180	6%	Melanoma of the skin	42,600
Kidney & renal pelvis	50,290	5%	Non-Hodgkin lymphoma	36,350
Non-Hodgkin lymphoma	44,120	4%	Thyroid	31,940
Oral cavity & pharynx	38,700	4%	Pancreas	29,240
Leukemia	35,810	4%	Kidney & renal pelvis	28,710
Pancreas	32,970	3%	Leukemia	24,840
All Sites	**983,160**	**100%**	**All Sites**	**934,870**

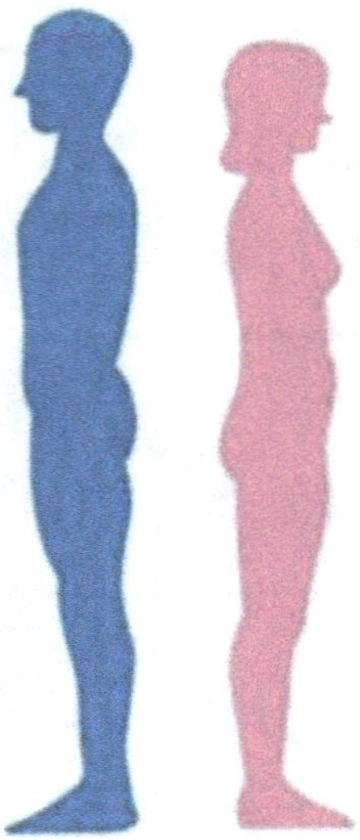

Research suggests that doctors will diagnose around 60,650 new cases of leukemia in the United States in 2022.

Around 16
cases pe
day!

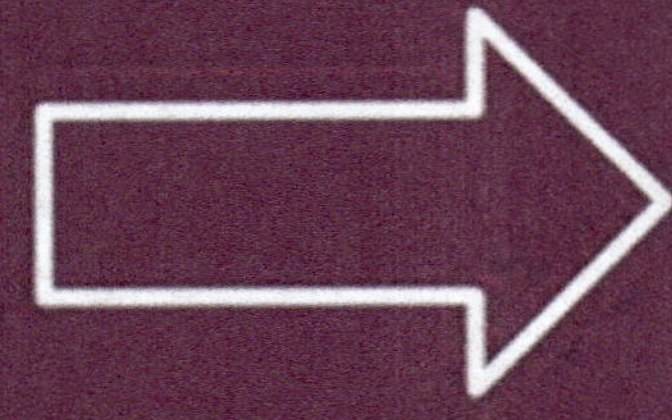

Unfortunately, an estimated 24,000 people will lose their battle with the disease.

Around
people p
day!

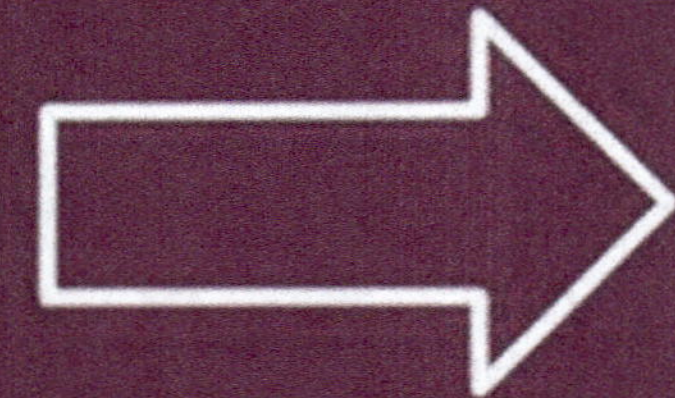

A leukemia diagnosis is definitely scary, but there are different treatment options to fight the cancer. Treatment depends on the type of leukemia, the stage of the disease, and the patient's overall health. Some treatments are:

Chemotherapy

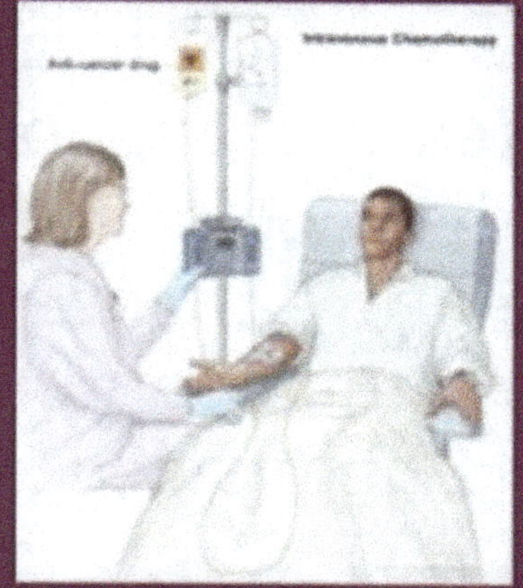

Immunotherapy

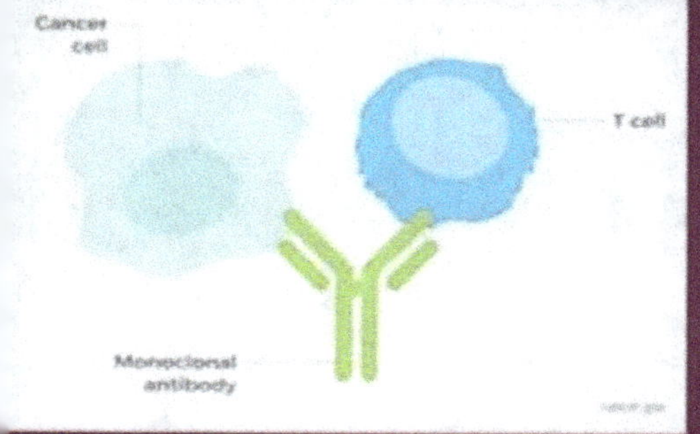

Bone Marrow Transplant

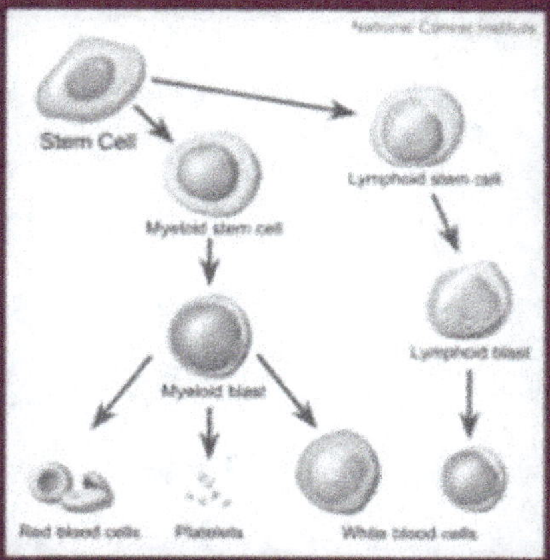

Clinical Trials

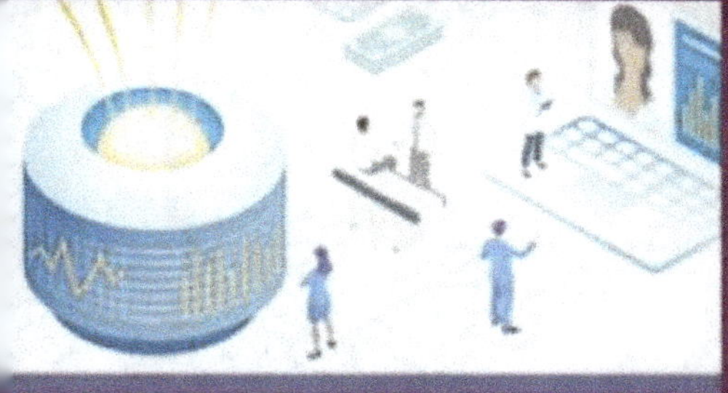

My grandma began treatment soon after her diagnosis. She chose a mixture of chemotherapy and medication at UPMC Shadyside Hospital.

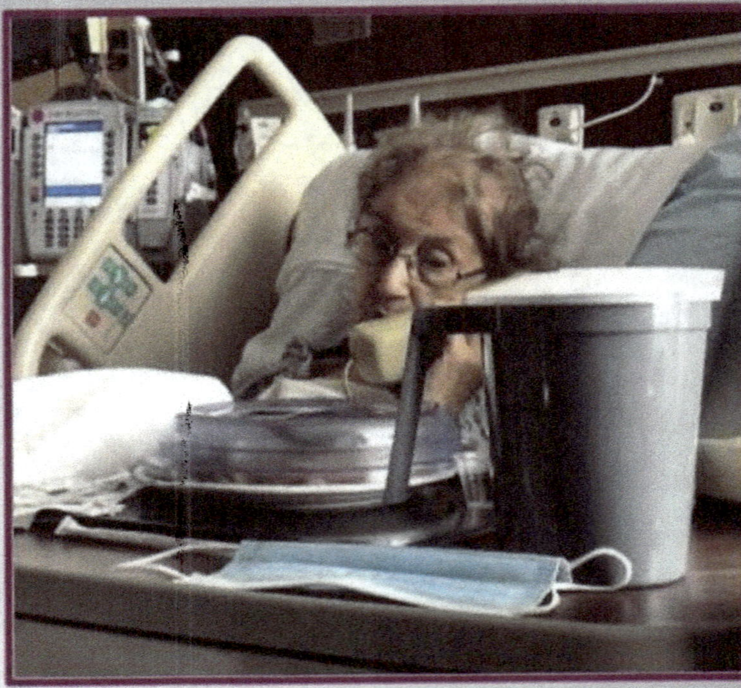

Officer Mark started on chemotherapy, which did help but he did not reach complete remission. Doctors switched him to immunotherapy with similar results. Finally, he received two stem cell transplants (one from a stranger and one from a relative) and took part in a clinical trial.

Chemotherapy is a cancer treatment that uses drugs and medications to treat cancer and/or symptoms. The drugs kill cancerous cells and block the formation of new ones. There are different types of chemotherapy, and patients decide with their doctor the kind of chemo right for them.
Some chemo options include:

Inpatient versus outpatient

By mouth versus by injection

Treatment cycle length versus rest period length

No matter the choices made, chemotherapy comes with side effects because the drugs are targeting the patient's own body. Sometimes healthy cells are targeted by mistake!

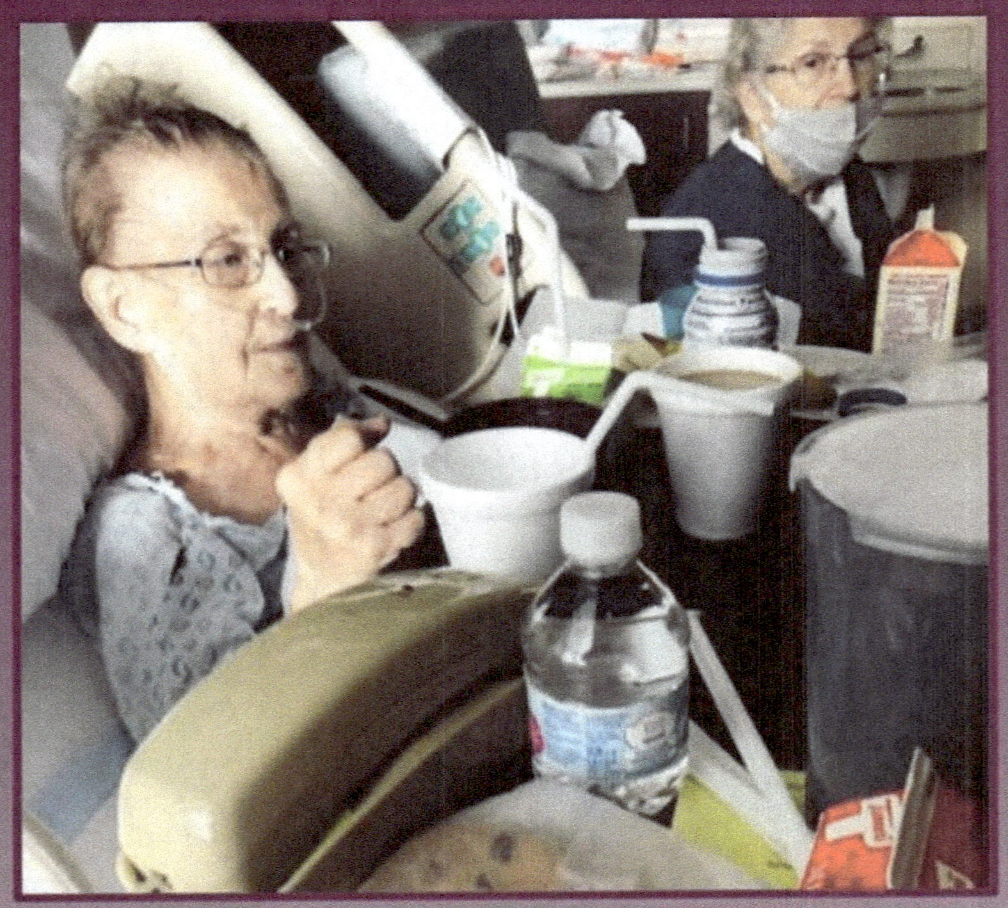

Chemotherapy occurs in cycles so the body can rest from side effects. Common side effects are fatigue, nausea, and hair loss. Other less common side effects are rashes and neuropathy.

Immunotherapy is different from chemotherapy because it uses the body's own immune system rather than drugs. It makes your immune system recognize cancer cells as bad and fight them, which slows or stops the spread. Immunotherapy treatment involves a shot of a biologic agent directly into a vein near the cancer. Patients receive the treatment for several weeks.

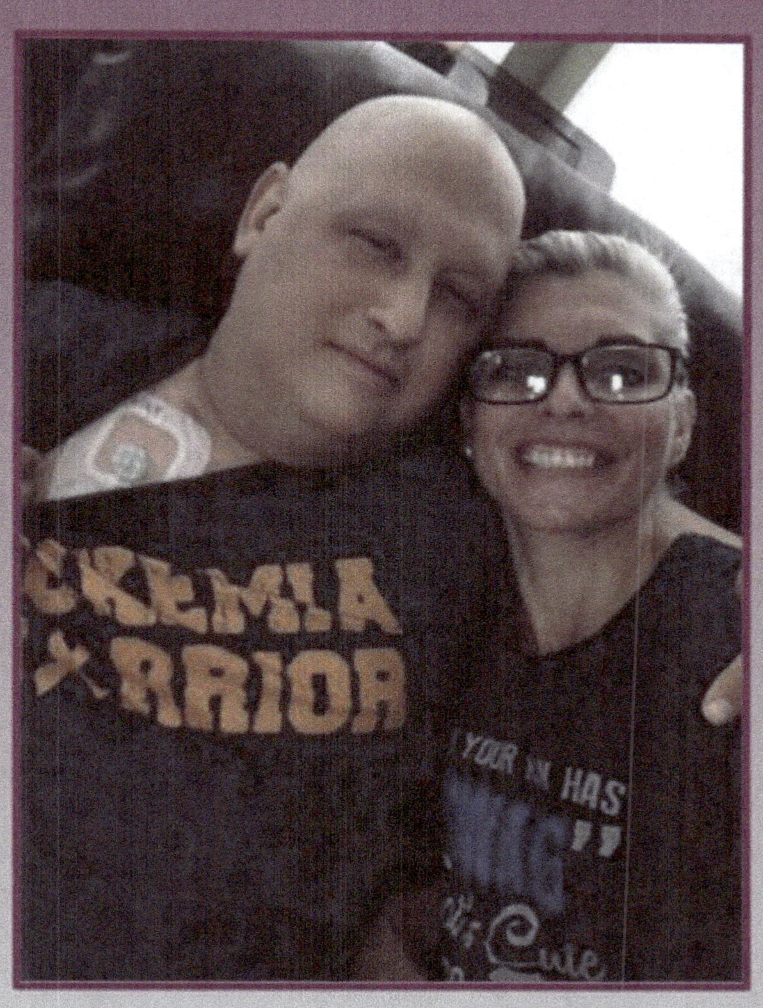

Immunotherapy uses biologic agents like cytokines, immunomodulators, monoclonal antibodies, and gene therapy. Each different agent has different side effects. A reaction at the injection site, headaches, muscle aches, fever, and weakness are some of the side effects a patient might have.

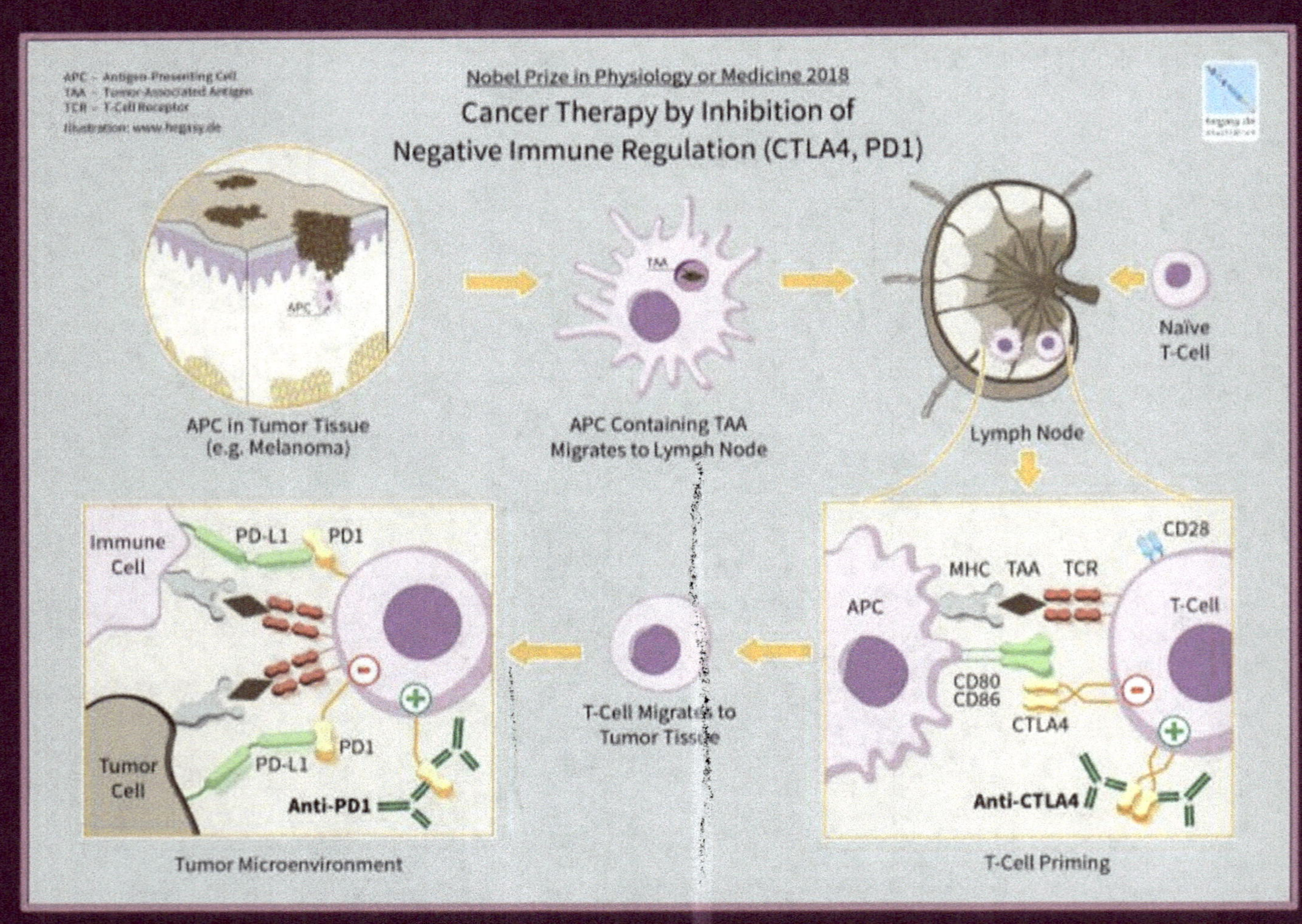

A bone marrow transplant is a special treatment to deal with cancer or other diseases. It involves taking stem cells from bone marrow, filtering them, and giving the healthy ones back to the patient. Transplants are performed by a peripheral intravenous injection. However, patients are at an increased risk of infection due to their disease. They may also experience side effects like nausea, fevers, and stomach problems. Officer Mark received two transplants because he relapsed after the first one.

In general, doctors refer patients to clinical trials when regular treatments fail. They are newer options found through research on animals that need to be tested on humans. Patients are very carefully watched to make sure they are safe!

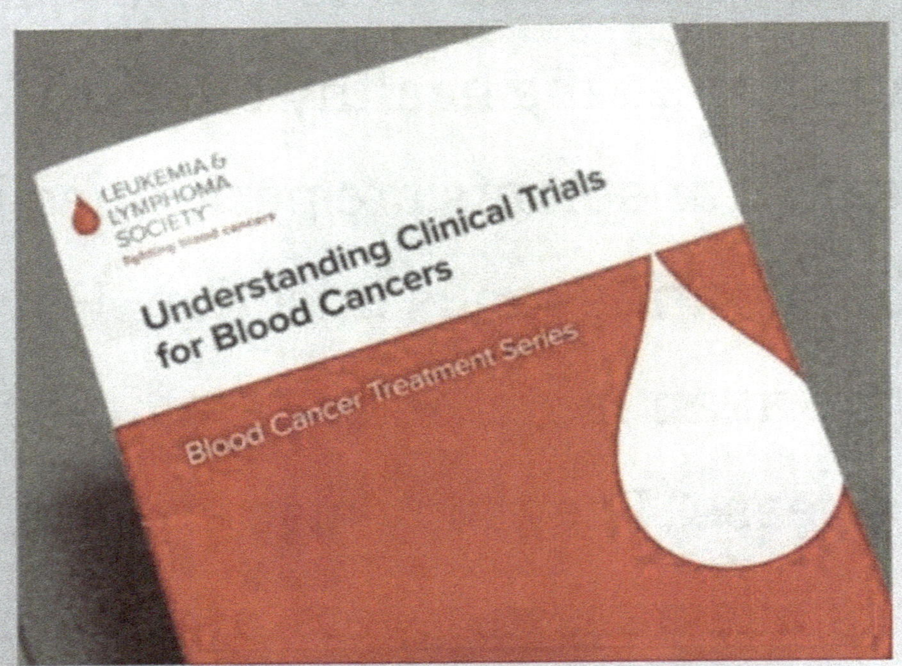

Officer Mark was in a clinical trial for Car-T treatment after his second stem cell treatment relapse. He was the third person in the world to receive that particular Car-T regiment.

Officer Mark has not technically reached remission. He is currently on a chemotherapy maintenance regiment.

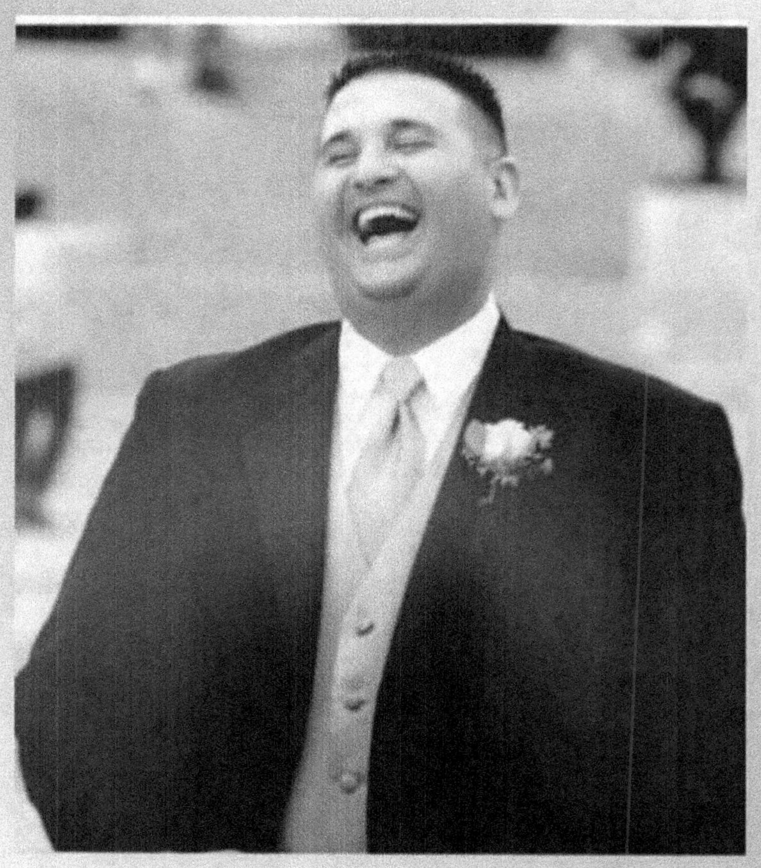

He takes chemo pills every day, a large dose once a week, and intravenous chemo once a month. Officer Mark remains optimistic.

My Great Gram was not reaching remission in the hospital. She was there for months before everyone decided she should go home to continue treatment. A nurse came to give her medications. It was nice to have her home with everyone.

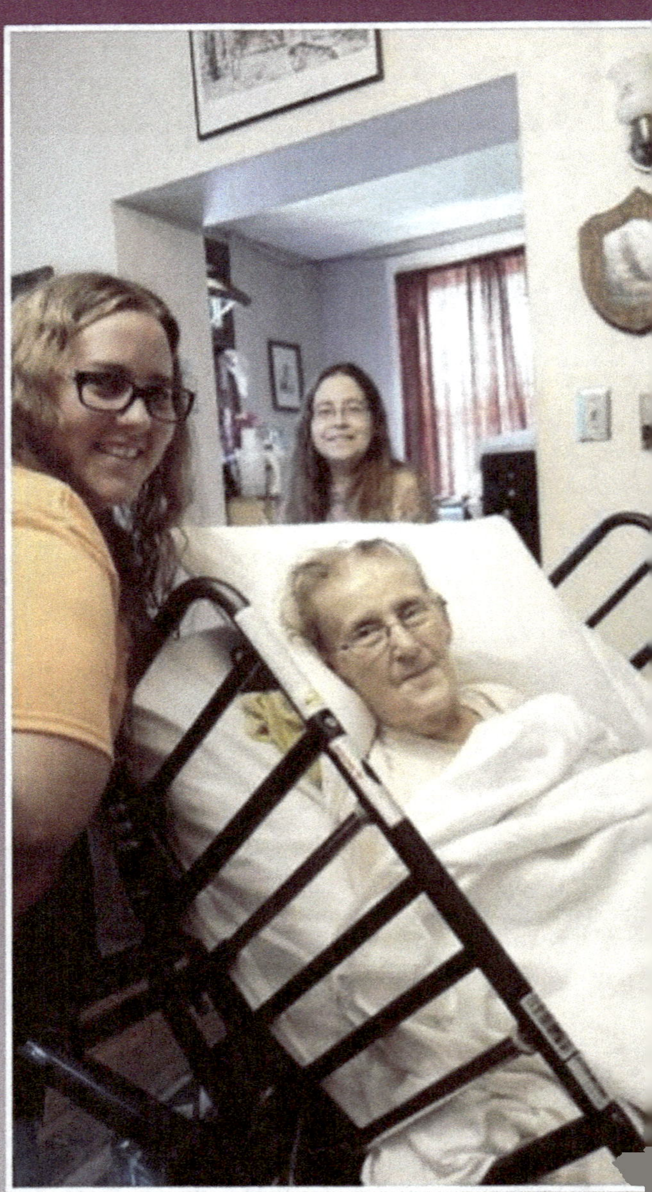

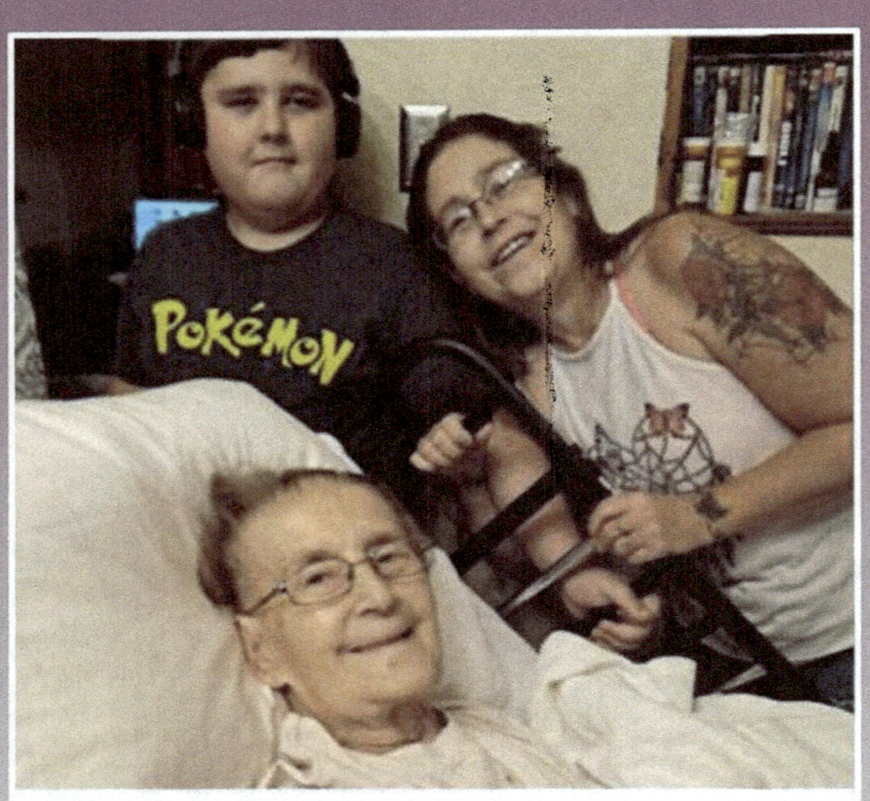

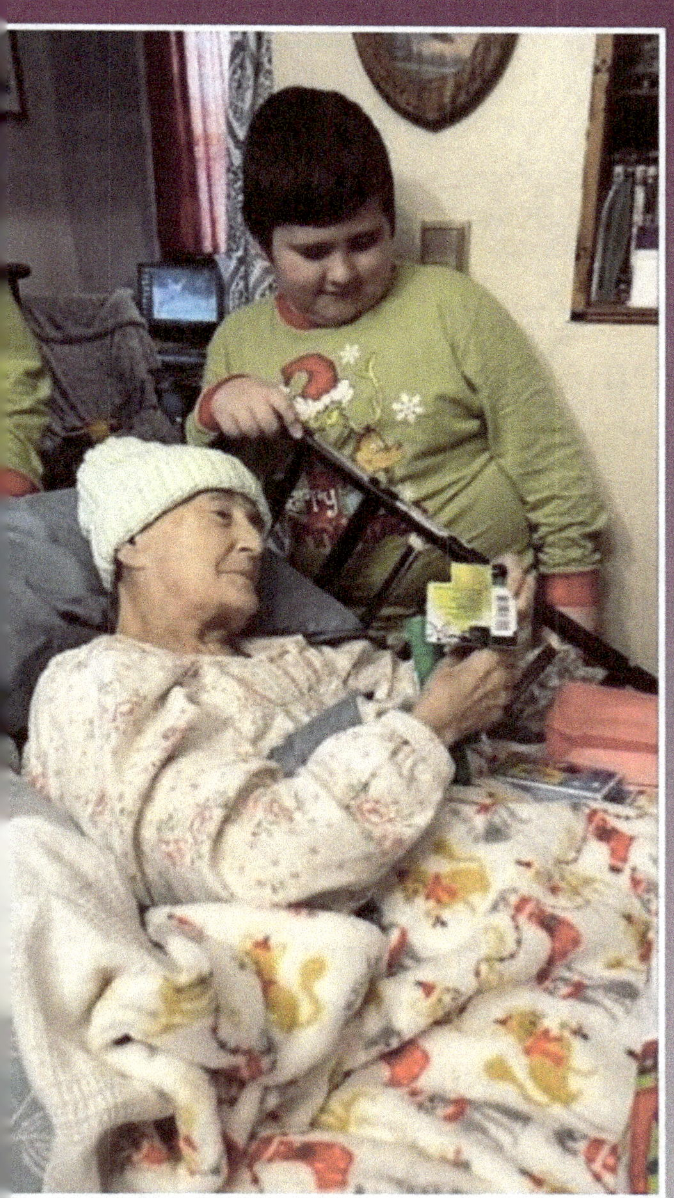

Unfortunately, she lost her battle with Leukemia December 30, 2020. She was home with family for the holidays and surrounded by love.

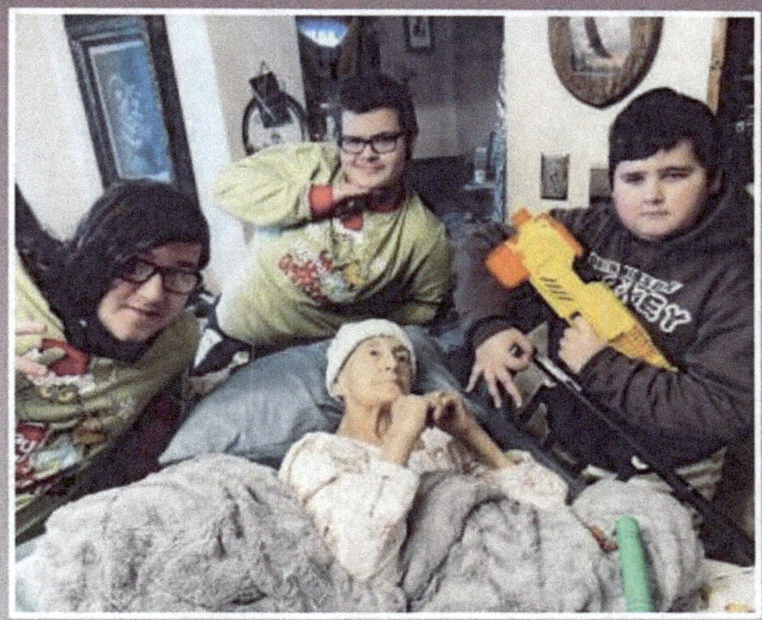

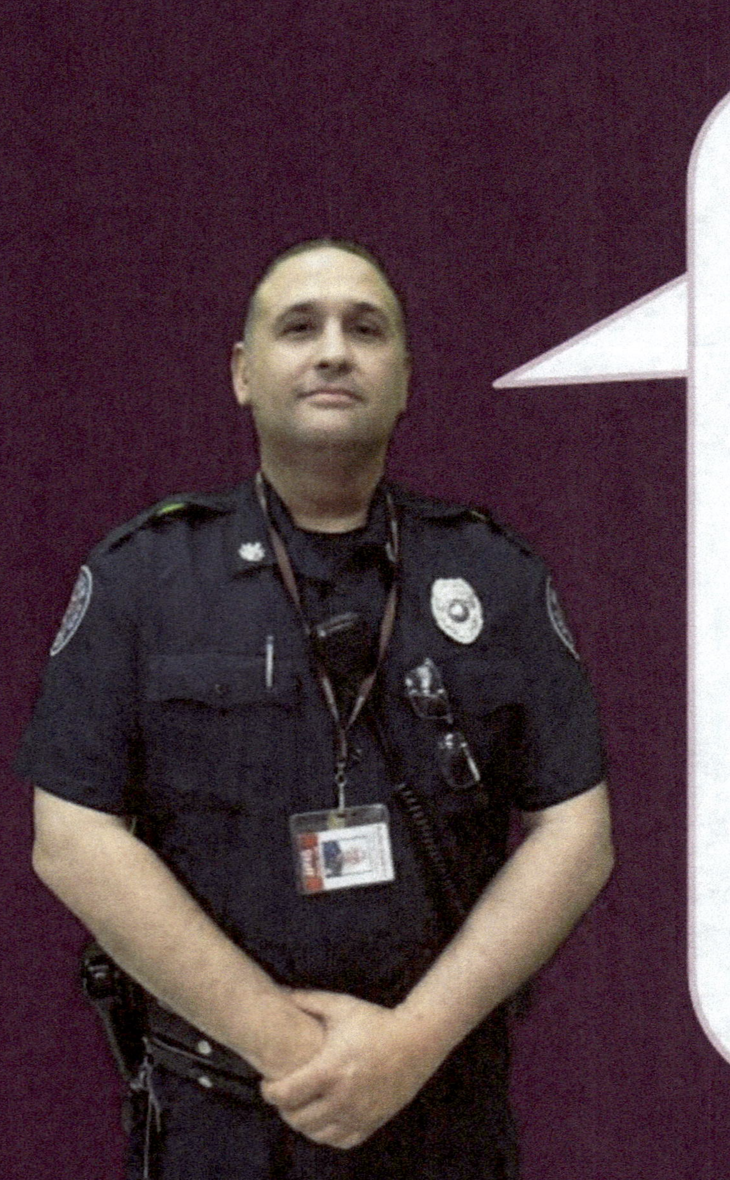

Leukemia is physically hard on patients. It is very tough emotionally as well. Officer Mark said this about his experience:
The emotions can be quite extreme... the financial burden is especially heavy, especially while in the hospital. During transplant, you're in isolation for up to 30 days and maybe allowed one visitor for a short period of time. When I was at U of Penn, I was in the hospital for 35 days, and in the midst of COVID. So no visitors were allowed. You just have to keep a positive attitude and convince yourself at some point you're going to beat the disease.

The financial and emotional burden also extends to a patient's loved ones. Officer Mark said how hard it was for his wife, and how she had to shoulder extra household responsibilities.

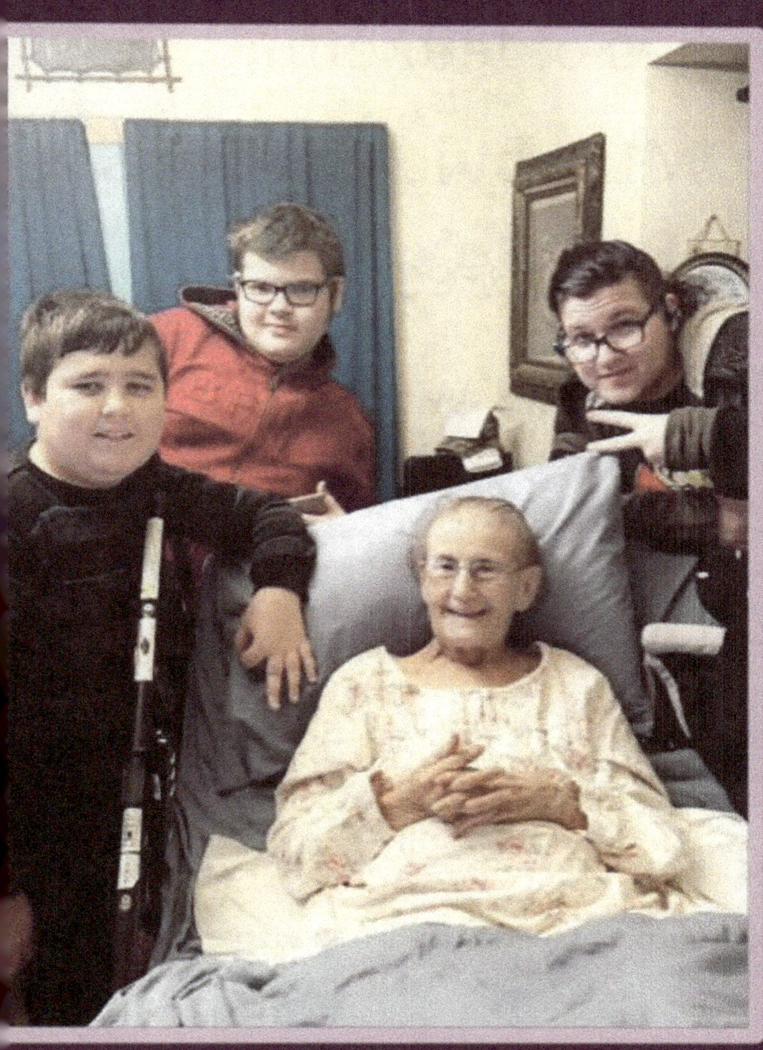

The emotions in my family were very strong. My Great Gram was always there for everyone in any way she could be. So having her need so much help and being away from family while she was in the hospital was really hard for everyone. She stayed strong for as long as she could.

Unfortunately there is still no cure for leukemia. Part of the reason for that is the many different types of leukemia. ALL, AML, CLL, and CML would all require their own specific cures. The subtypes of those four kinds would also need their own cures. Scientists therefore focus on curing a specific type of leukemia, rather than curing leukemia as a whole.

But there has been some success! Acute Promyelocytic Leukemia is a type of Myeloid Lleukemia that has over a 90% cure rate! Researchers discovered a unique and successful Vitamin A treatment that effectively cures this specific leukemia. As we do more research into other types of leukemia, we will surely figure out how to cure them, too!

Vocabulary

Remission - A decrease or disappearance of signs and
symptoms of a disease.

Neuropathy - Weakness, numbness, and pain from nerve
damage, usually in the hands and feet.

Inpatient - A patient who stays in the hospital for treatmer

Outpatient - A patient who does not stay in the hospital for
treatment

Stem Cells - Stem cells are special human cells that have t
ability to develop into many different cell types,
from muscle cells to brain cells.

Biologic - A substance made from a living organism or its
products

Intravenous Injection - A shot inserted directly into the ve:

Car-T Treatment - Harvesting a patient's own cells and
genetically engineering them to target
cancer cells.

Leukemia (or any kind of cancer) can be a scary diagnosis, but anyone who gets that diagnosis should stay positive and fight as hard as they can. In Pittsburgh alone there are so many different teams of doctors working to help cure every kind of cancer!

From the Allegheny Health Network to UPMC, it is inspiring to see all the research and support going into battling this disease. I hope this book inspires people and helps with the fight.

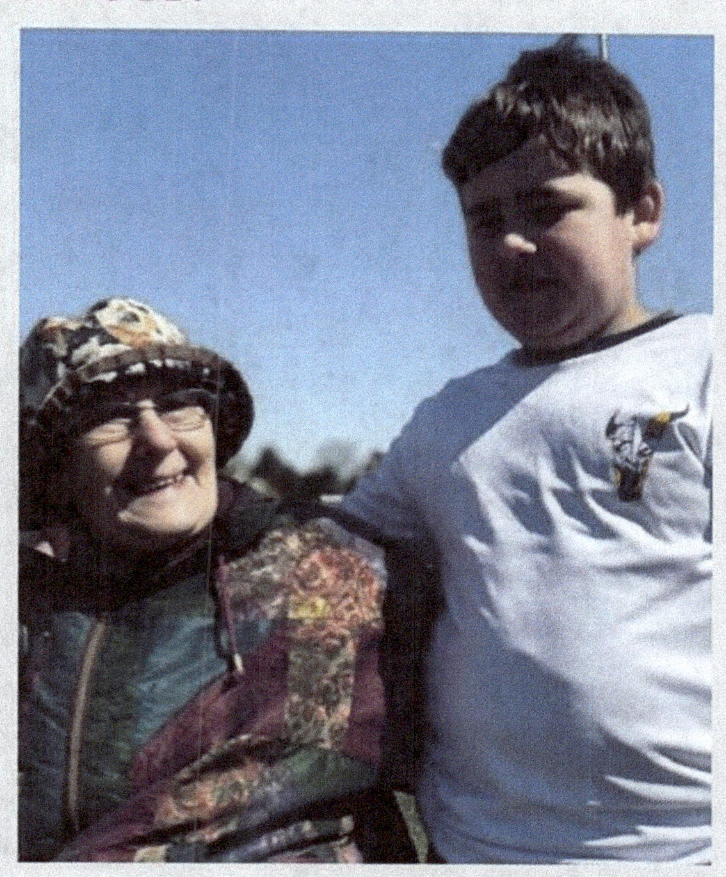

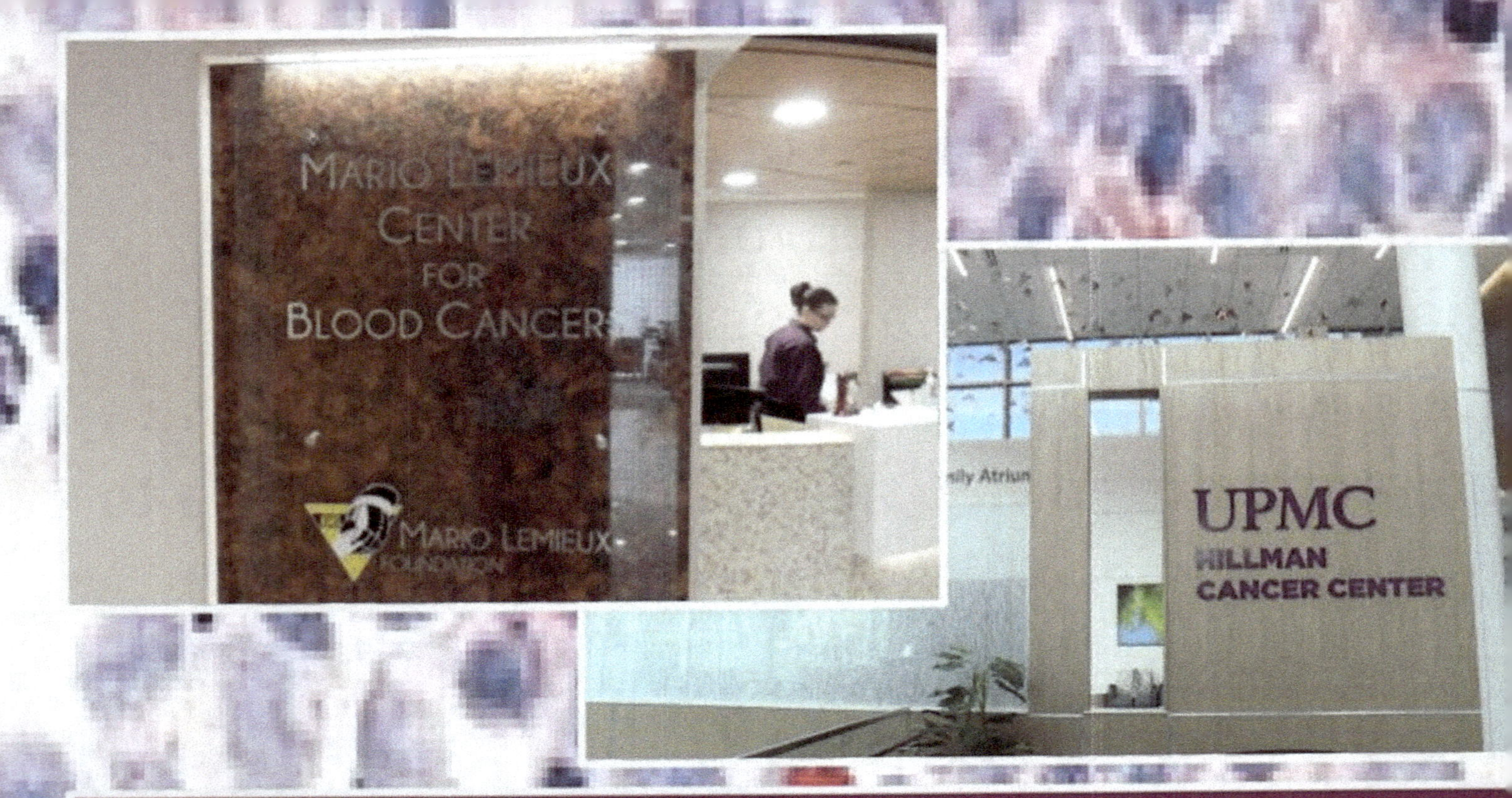

UPMC Hillman Cancer Center is a designated comprehensive cancer center with over 70 locations in Pennsylvania and some surrounding states. The Mario Lemeiux Center for Blood Cancers, located in Pittsburgh, provides research-driven care to patients with leukemia and other blood cancers. It is always up to date on the newest treatments and research, and offers collaborative care as part of the UPMC network. The Center also provides numerous supportive services to patients and their loved ones, including behavioral medicine, nutrition for blood cancer, pain management, social support, and more. You can visit https://hillman.upmc.com/difference/supporting to find other ways to donate or volunteer.

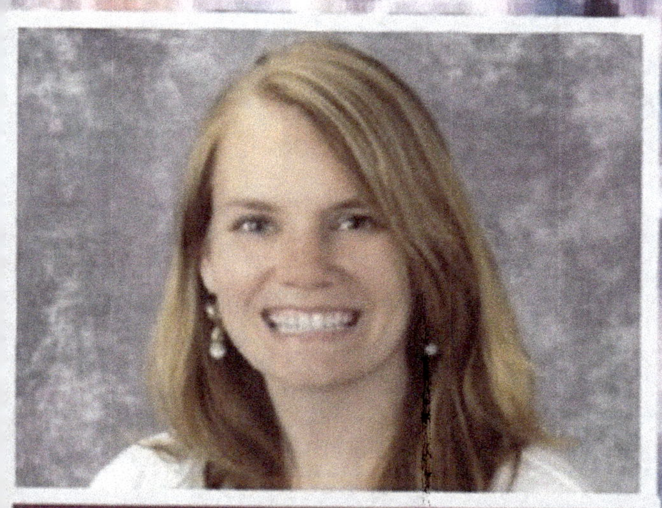

Dr. Kelly Bailey

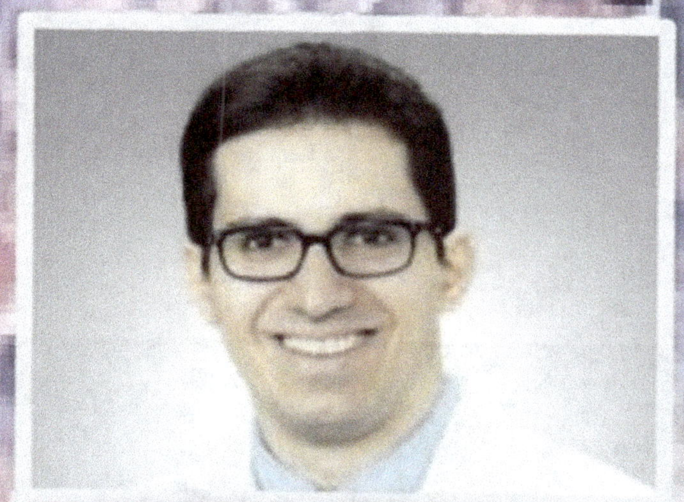

Dr. Konstantinos Lontos

I want to specially thank two doctors who volunteered their time to help me complete this book. Their assistance in understanding the science and explaining things in a way I could understand helped a lot.

Kelly M. Bailey, MD, PhD is a pediatric oncologist and physician-scientist who helped me understand the types of leukemia and the journey toward a cure.

Konstantinos Lontos, MD is an internist who specializes in medical oncology and hematology oncology. He helped me understand the types, symptoms, and treatments of leukemia.

I would also like to thank Dr. Taofeek Owonikoko, Dr. Annie Im, and Dr. Margaret Rosenzweig for their contributions and connections. I could not have done this without all of them.

Dr. Ellen Cavanaugh

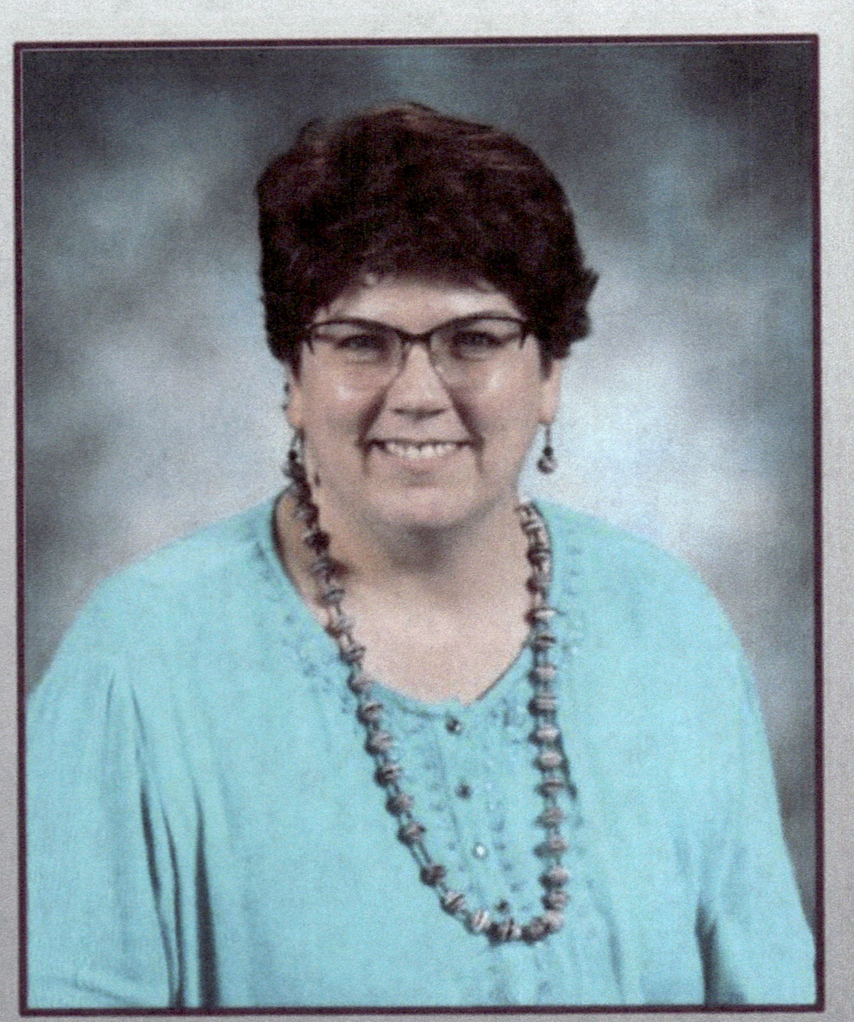

Dr. Ellen spent countless hours helping students with their projec[ts] in the BACS Media Lab. She was supportive, and was never afraid t[o] push her students to make sure they met their goals. She founded the Media Lab and also Grow a Generation. She taught students how to use technology, conduct research properly, and to speak up to professionals. Without Dr. Ellen at Baden Academy we would have missed out on so many great idea[s] innovations, and popcorn though[ts] I'm thankful I got the chance to work with Dr. Ellen and she was there to believe in me and help m[e] start writing this book.

Thank you Dr. Ellen Cavanaugh

Great Gram Dedication Page

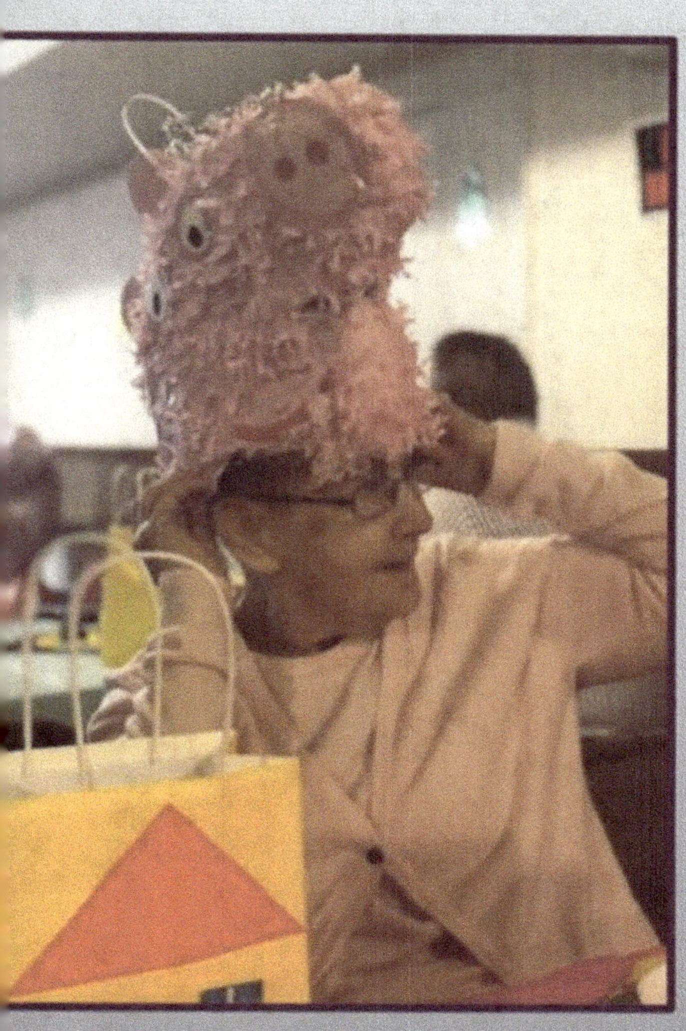

My Great Gram helped our family by spending countless hours cleaning and cooking. She was very supportive. She loved to bake and we loved to eat her famous little boy gingerbread cookies. Great Gram was always ready to come over and help anytime we needed her to be there. Even after she was diagnosed she was still in good spirits and was as energetic as she could be. She still danced in her bed and asked us how we were doing and what fun we were having when we visited every day. She was an amazing Great Gram and I miss her very much.

Thank you Great Gram

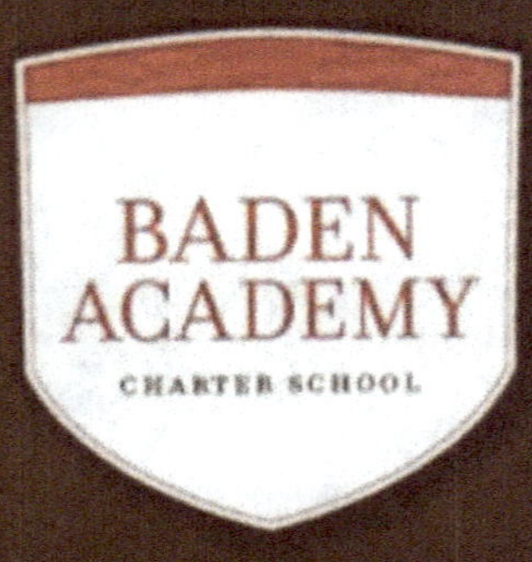

Baden Academy Charter School

This public charter school in Western PA works to inspire personal excellence. They cultivate the inherent gifts and talents present in all children by providing a curriculum that integrates the arts and sciences in a highly interactive, hands-on environment.

Grow a Generation

Grow a Generation partners with gifted and talented young people and teachers to make meaningful projects possible. Faculty, students, and student teams apply in their school to be accepted into the fellowship program. Once selected, they embark on a year-long odyssey to publish a book, create a digital artifact, or enter a STEM competition. Find out more at growageneration.com

9 781716 401596